THYROID CANCER

DIET

COOKBOOK

FOR BEGINNERS

The Ultimate Guide with 20 Quick & Easy Recipes for Hypothyroidism and Hashimoto's Relief

Patricia Camire

Copyright © 2023 by Patricia Camire

CHECK OTHER BOOKS BY AUTHOR:

TABLE OF CONTENT

INTRODUCTION 5

CHAPTER ONE 6

GENERAL OVERVIEW OF THYROID CANCER 6

The Thyroid Gland and Its Functions 6

Common Thyroid Disorders 7

Thyroid Cancer: Understanding the Intricacies..................... 8

Hypothyroidism: The Sleeping Thyroid 8

Hashimoto's Disease: An Autoimmune Symphony................ 9

The Effect of Nutrition on Thyroid Function......................... 9

Foods to Support Thyroid Health 10

Foods to Avoid.. 11

Navigating the Thyroid Terrain: A Holistic Approach......... 11

CHAPTER TWO 13

DELICIOUS THYROID CANCER DIET RECIPES 13

1. Grilled Salmon with Lemon-Dill Quinoa 13

2. Roasted Turkey and Sweet Potato Salad.......................... 14

3. Quinoa-Stuffed Bell Peppers with Avocado Salsa 16

4. Spinach and Chickpea Salad with Lemon-Tahini Dressing
.... 17

5. Lentil and Vegetable Soup 19

6. Baked Cod with Quinoa and Roasted Vegetables 20

7. Quinoa and Kale Stuffed Bell Peppers 22

8. Chicken and Vegetable Stir-Fry with Brown Rice 23

9. Quinoa and Chickpea Salad with Lemon-Turmeric Dressing 25

10. Shrimp and Vegetable Skewers with Quinoa 26

11. Turkey and Sweet Potato Chili 27

12. Quinoa and Broccoli Casserole 29

13. Egg and Vegetable Breakfast Wrap 30

14. Lentil and Vegetable Curry 31

15. Greek Chicken Salad with Quinoa 33

16. Salmon and Asparagus Foil Packets 34

17. Quinoa and Black Bean Salad with Avocado-Lime Dressing 35

18. Turkey and Vegetable Skillet with Cauliflower Rice 36

19. Veggie-Packed Quinoa Bowl with Lemon-Tahini Dressing 38

20. Chicken and Vegetable Kabobs with Herb Marinade 39

CONCLUSION 42

INTRODUCTION

A subtle revolution unfolded in the quiet corners of Sarah's kitchen with the arrival of the "Thyroid Cancer Diet Cookbook for Beginners."

When she was dealing with the aftermath of thyroid cancer, she found comfort in its pages. The cookbook, which served as a guiding light throughout her recovery, transformed her daily meals into a healing symphony.

Sarah experienced renewed vitality and balance after trying each thyroid-friendly recipe. The nutrient-dense dishes not only nourished her body but also lifted her spirits, providing solace from the difficulties of post-cancer life.

As she savoured the flavorful concoctions, Sarah realised that this cookbook was more than just ingredients; it was a beacon of hope, a companion on her journey to reclaiming health and rediscovering joy with each bite.

CHAPTER ONE

GENERAL OVERVIEW OF THYROID CANCER

The thyroid gland, which is butterfly-shaped and located at the base of the neck, regulates our body's metabolism.

This intricate endocrine powerhouse controls the production and release of hormones that affect nearly every cell, including energy levels and temperature regulation.

As we delve into the complex landscape of thyroid health, we will look at not only the essential functions of this gland, but also the shadows cast by thyroid disorders, with a particular emphasis on Thyroid Cancer, a formidable adversary.

The Thyroid Gland and Its Functions

The thyroid gland, located at the centre of the endocrine system, secretes hormones, primarily thyroxine (T4) and triiodothyronine (T3), which act as messengers and regulate metabolism and growth. This intricate dance of hormones maintains a delicate balance by influencing heart rate, weight, and temperature.

Consider the thyroid as a conductor, orchestrating the harmonious symphony of our physiological processes.

When this symphony fails, disruptions reverberate throughout the body. Thyroid hormones control the rate at which cells convert nutrients into energy, which influences the speed of bodily functions.

Thyroid hormones keep the body's cells in balance, which is essential for overall health. From the vigour of youth to the graceful ageing of old age, the thyroid is a constant maestro orchestrating the rhythm of life.

Common Thyroid Disorders

Various disorders can disrupt the delicate ballet of thyroid function's smooth performance. Among them, Thyroid Cancer strikes a poignant note—a diagnosis that reverberates throughout many people's lives.

However, it is not alone in this story; hypothyroidism and Hashimoto's disease also appear, each with their own set of challenges.

Thyroid Cancer: Understanding the Intricacies

Thyroid cancer occurs when the cells of the thyroid gland grow abnormally. While it accounts for a small percentage of cancer diagnoses, the impact is significant.

Symptoms may include a lump or swelling in the neck, persistent hoarseness, difficulty swallowing, or vocal changes. While exact causes are unknown, genetics, radiation exposure, and pre-existing thyroid conditions may all play a role.

Hypothyroidism: The Sleeping Thyroid

Hypothyroidism, on the other hand, refers to an underactive thyroid gland that does not produce enough hormones. Fatigue, weight gain, cold intolerance, and depression may occur. Hypothyroidism's insidious nature often results in a delayed diagnosis, but early intervention is critical to avoiding complications.

Hashimoto's Disease: An Autoimmune Symphony

Hashimoto's, an autoimmune disorder, develops when the body mistakenly attacks thyroid tissue. This relentless assault causes inflammation, reducing the thyroid's ability to produce hormones.

Fatigue, weight gain, and muscle weakness are common symptoms. Understanding the complex interactions between genetics and the immune system is critical for navigating this autoimmune symphony.

The Effect of Nutrition on Thyroid Function

Adequate nutrition lays the foundation for optimal thyroid function. Key nutrients—iodine, selenium, zinc, and omega-3 fatty acids—are the unsung heroes ensuring the thyroid's smooth operation. Iodine, a crucial component of thyroid hormones, is derived from dietary sources like seafood and iodized salt.

Selenium, found in nuts, seeds, and poultry, protects the thyroid from oxidative damage. Zinc, abundant in meat, nuts, and whole grains, supports hormone production.

Meanwhile, omega-3 fatty acids, present in fatty fish and flaxseeds, mitigate inflammation, a common denominator in thyroid disorders.

However, a delicate balance is essential, as excessive amounts can tip the scales. Iodine excess, for instance, may paradoxically lead to thyroid dysfunction. Striking this balance through a well-rounded diet is paramount.

Foods to Support Thyroid Health

A thyroid-friendly diet revolves around whole, nutrient-dense foods. Fruits and vegetables, rich in antioxidants, serve as guardians against inflammation.

Lean proteins, such as poultry, fish, and legumes, offer essential amino acids crucial for hormone synthesis. Whole grains and nuts provide the necessary nutrients for overall well-being. Integrating these foods into one's diet fosters an environment conducive to thyroid health.

Antioxidants play a pivotal role, countering oxidative stress that may compromise thyroid function. Berries, leafy greens, and nuts are potent sources, serving as allies in the battle against inflammation—a common precursor to thyroid disorders.

Foods to Avoid

Just as certain foods support thyroid health, others warrant caution. Goitrogens, substances that may interfere with thyroid function, are found in certain cruciferous vegetables like broccoli, cabbage, and kale.

While these foods can be part of a balanced diet, cooking or steaming reduces their goitrogenic potential.

Excessive intake of iodine-rich foods, such as seaweed and iodine supplements, may interrupt thyroid function. Striking a balance is crucial to prevent unintended consequences.

Navigating the Thyroid Terrain: A Holistic Approach

Understanding the complexities of thyroid health involves unraveling the symphony of hormonal interplay.

Whether facing Thyroid Cancer, Hypothyroidism, or Hashimoto's, a multidimensional approach is essential.

Nutrition serves as a linchpin, offering a tangible means to support thyroid function.

As we traverse the intricate terrain of thyroid health, a harmonious symphony emerges—one where awareness, nutrition, and medical guidance converge.

This is not merely a journey through the anatomy of a gland; it is an exploration of the interconnected rhythms that sustain life, where every nutrient, every morsel, becomes a note in the melody of well-being.

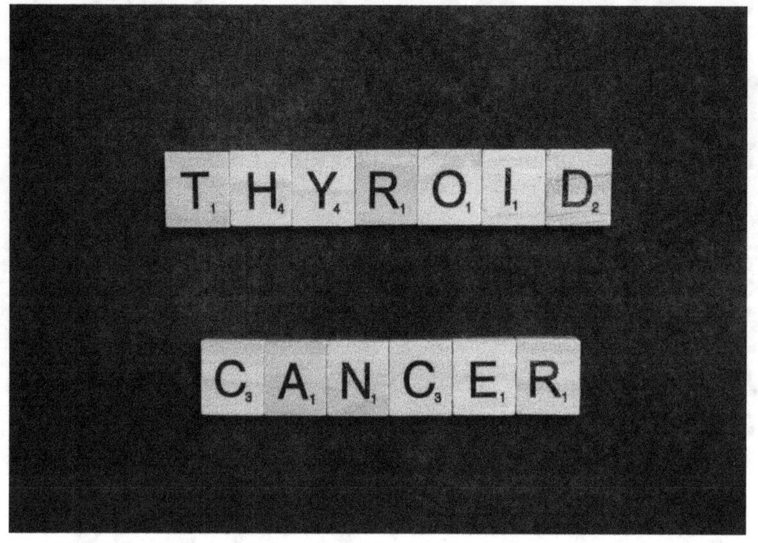

CHAPTER TWO

DELICIOUS THYROID CANCER DIET RECIPES

1. Grilled Salmon with Lemon-Dill Quinoa

Ingredients:

- 4 salmon fillets

- 1 cup quinoa, rinsed

- 2 cups vegetable broth

- Zest and juice of 1 lemon

- 2 tablespoons fresh dill, chopped

- 2 tablespoons olive oil

- Salt and pepper to taste

- Mixed vegetables for grilling (zucchini, cherry tomatoes, bell peppers)

Instructions:

1. Preheat the grill.

2. Season salmon fillets with salt, pepper, and a drizzle of olive oil.

3. Grill salmon for 4-5 minutes per side or until cooked through.

4. In a saucepan, bring vegetable broth to a boil. Add quinoa, reduce heat, and simmer for 15-20 minutes until cooked.

5. Fluff the quinoa with a fork and stir in lemon zest, lemon juice, chopped dill, and a drizzle of olive oil.

6. Grill mixed vegetables until tender.

7. Serve grilled salmon over lemon-dill quinoa, with grilled vegetables on the side.

2. Roasted Turkey and Sweet Potato Salad

Ingredients:

- 1 pound of cooked and shredded turkey breast

- 2 sweet potatoes, peeled and diced

- 1 tablespoon olive oil

- 1 teaspoon smoked paprika

- 1 teaspoon cumin

- Salt and pepper to taste

- Mixed salad greens (spinach, arugula, or kale)

- 1/4 cup cranberries (dried or fresh)

- 1/4 cup pumpkin seeds

- Balsamic vinaigrette dressing

Instructions:

1. Preheat the oven to 400°F (200°C).

2. Toss diced sweet potatoes with olive oil, smoked paprika, cumin, salt, and pepper.

3. Roast sweet potatoes in the oven for 20-25 minutes until tender.

4. In a large bowl, combine shredded turkey, roasted sweet potatoes, mixed salad greens, cranberries, and pumpkin seeds.

5. Drizzle with balsamic vinaigrette dressing and toss to combine.

6. Serve the roasted turkey and sweet potato salad as a nutritious and flavorful meal.

3. Quinoa-Stuffed Bell Peppers with Avocado Salsa

Ingredients:

- 4 halved and seeds removed bell peppers

- 1 cup quinoa, cooked

- 1 can (15 oz) of drained and rinsed black beans,

- 1 cup of fresh or frozen corn kernels

- 1 cup cherry tomatoes, diced

- 1/2 red onion, finely chopped

- 1 avocado, diced

- Juice of 2 limes

- 2 tablespoons fresh cilantro, chopped

- Salt and pepper to taste

- Optional: Shredded chicken for added protein

Instructions:

1. Preheat the oven to 375°F (190°C).

2. In a large bowl, combine cooked quinoa, black beans, corn, cherry tomatoes, and red onion.

3. In a separate bowl, mix diced avocado, lime juice, chopped cilantro, salt, and pepper to make the salsa.

4. Stuff each bell pepper half with the quinoa mixture. If desired, add shredded chicken on top.

5. Bake in the oven for 25-30 minutes or until the peppers are tender.

6. Top each stuffed pepper with avocado salsa before serving.

4. Spinach and Chickpea Salad with Lemon-Tahini Dressing

Ingredients:

- 4 cups fresh spinach leaves

- 1 can (15 oz) of drained and rinsed chickpeas,

- 1 cucumber, diced

- 1 cup cherry tomatoes, halved

- 1/4 cup red onion, finely chopped

- 1/4 cup feta cheese, crumbled (optional)

- 2 tablespoons olive oil

- 1 tablespoon tahini

- Juice of 1 lemon

- 1 clove garlic, minced

- Salt and pepper to taste

Instructions:

1. In a large bowl, combine fresh spinach, chickpeas, diced cucumber, cherry tomatoes, and red onion.

2. In a small bowl, whisk together olive oil, tahini, lemon juice, minced garlic, salt, and pepper to make the dressing.

3. Drizzle the dressing over the salad and toss to coat.

4. If desired, sprinkle crumbled feta cheese over the top before serving.

5. Lentil and Vegetable Soup

Ingredients:

- 1 cup dried green or brown lentils, rinsed

- 1 onion, diced

- 2 carrots, peeled and chopped

- 2 celery stalks, chopped

- 3 cloves garlic, minced

- 1 can (14 oz) diced tomatoes

- 6 cups vegetable broth

- 1 teaspoon ground cumin

- 1 teaspoon smoked paprika

- Salt and pepper to taste

- Fresh parsley for garnish

Instructions:

1. In a large pot, sauté diced onion, carrots, and celery until softened.

2. Add minced garlic, ground cumin, and smoked paprika to the pot, stirring to combine.

3. Pour in vegetable broth and add lentils and diced tomatoes. Make sure it boil, then reduce heat and simmer for 25-30 minutes or until lentils are tender.

4. Season the soup with salt and pepper make it sweet.

5. Garnish with fresh parsley before serving.

6. Baked Cod with Quinoa and Roasted Vegetables

Ingredients:

- 4 cod fillets

- 1 cup quinoa, cooked

- 1 zucchini, sliced

- 1 bell pepper, diced

- 1 cup cherry tomatoes, halved

- 2 tablespoons olive oil

- 1 teaspoon dried oregano

- 1 teaspoon garlic powder

- Salt and pepper to taste

- Lemon wedges for serving

Instructions:

1. Preheat the oven to 400°F (200°C).

2. Place cod fillets on a baking sheet lined with parchment paper.

3. In a bowl, mix sliced zucchini, diced bell pepper, and cherry tomatoes with olive oil, dried oregano, garlic powder, salt, and pepper.

4. Spread the vegetable mixture around the cod fillets.

5. Bake for 15-20 minutes or until the cod is flaky and cooked through.

6. Serve the baked cod over a bed of cooked quinoa, with lemon wedges on the side.

7. Quinoa and Kale Stuffed Bell Peppers

Ingredients:

- 4 halved and seeds removed bell peppers

- 1 cup quinoa, cooked

- 2 cups kale, finely chopped

- 1 can (15 oz) of drained and rinsed black beans,

- 1 cup of fresh or frozen corn kernels

- 1 teaspoon cumin

- 1 teaspoon chili powder

- Salt and pepper to taste

- Salsa for topping (optional)

Instructions:

1. Preheat the oven to 375°F (190°C).

2. In a large bowl, combine cooked quinoa, chopped kale, black beans, corn, cumin, chili powder, salt, and pepper.

3. Put in each bell pepper half with the quinoa mixture.

4. Bake in the oven for 25-30 minutes or until the peppers are tender.

5. Top with salsa if desired before serving.

8. Chicken and Vegetable Stir-Fry with Brown Rice

Ingredients:

- 1 pound boneless, skinless chicken breasts, sliced

- 2 tablespoons soy sauce (low-sodium)

- 1 tablespoon oyster sauce

- 1 tablespoon sesame oil

- 1 tablespoon cornstarch

- 2 tablespoons vegetable oil

- 2 bell peppers, sliced

- 1 cup broccoli florets

- 1 carrot, julienned

- 3 green onions, sliced

- 2 cups cooked brown rice

Instructions:

1. In a bowl, mix sliced chicken with soy sauce, oyster sauce, sesame oil, and cornstarch. Let it marinate for 15-20 minutes.

2. Increase vegetable oil temperature in a wok or large skillet over high heat.

3. Stir-fry marinated chicken until cooked through. Take it out from the wok and set aside.

4. In the same wok, add more oil if needed and stir-fry bell peppers, broccoli, carrot, and green onions until crisp-tender.

5. Return the cooked chicken to the wok and toss everything together.

6. Serve the chicken and vegetable stir-fry over cooked brown rice.

9. Quinoa and Chickpea Salad with Lemon-Turmeric Dressing

Ingredients:

- 1 cup quinoa, cooked

- 1 can (15 oz) of drained and rinsed chickpeas

- 1 cucumber, diced

- 1 cup cherry tomatoes, halved

- 1/4 cup red onion, finely chopped

- 1/4 cup fresh parsley, chopped

- 2 tablespoons olive oil

- Juice of 1 lemon

- 1 teaspoon ground turmeric

- Salt and pepper to taste

Instructions:

1. In a large bowl, combine cooked quinoa, chickpeas, diced cucumber, cherry tomatoes, red onion, and fresh parsley.

2. In a small bowl, whisk together olive oil, lemon juice, ground turmeric, salt, and pepper to make the dressing.

3. Drizzle the dressing over the salad and toss to combine.

4. Refrigerate for at least 30 minutes before serving to let the flavors meld.

10. Shrimp and Vegetable Skewers with Quinoa

Ingredients:

- 1 pound large shrimp, peeled and deveined

- 2 bell peppers, cut into chunks

- 1 zucchini, sliced

- 1 red onion, cut into wedges

- 2 tablespoons olive oil

- 1 teaspoon dried thyme

- 1 teaspoon garlic powder

- Salt and pepper to taste

- 1 cup quinoa, cooked

- Lemon wedges for serving

Instructions:

1. Preheat the grill or oven.

2. In a bowl, toss shrimp, bell peppers, zucchini, and red onion with olive oil, dried thyme, garlic powder, salt, and pepper.

3. Thread shrimp and vegetables onto skewers.

4. Grill or bake for 8-10 minutes until shrimp are opaque and vegetables are tender.

5. Serve the skewers over a bed of cooked quinoa, with lemon wedges for a burst of freshness.

11. Turkey and Sweet Potato Chili

Ingredients:

- 1 pound ground turkey

- 2 sweet potatoes, peeled and diced

- 1 can (15 oz) of drained and rinsed black beans

- 1 can (15 oz) diced tomatoes

- 1 cup chicken or vegetable broth

- 1 onion, diced

- 2 cloves garlic, minced

- 1 tablespoon chili powder

- 1 teaspoon cumin

- Salt and pepper to taste

- Avocado slices and fresh cilantro for garnish

Instructions:

1. In a large pot, brown ground turkey over medium heat.

2. Add diced sweet potatoes, black beans, diced tomatoes, chicken or vegetable broth, diced onion, minced garlic, chili powder, cumin, salt, and pepper.

3. Bring to a simmer and let it cook for 20-25 minutes until sweet potatoes are tender.

4. Adjust seasoning to taste.

5. Serve the turkey and sweet potato chili topped with avocado slices and fresh cilantro.

12. Quinoa and Broccoli Casserole

Ingredients:

- 1 cup quinoa, uncooked

- 2 cups broccoli florets

- 1 cup shredded chicken breast (pre-cooked)

- 1/2 cup plain Greek yogurt

- 1/2 cup milk (dairy or plant-based)

- 1 cup shredded cheddar cheese

- 1 teaspoon Dijon mustard

- Salt and pepper to taste

- Panko breadcrumbs for topping (optional)

Instructions:

1. Preheat the oven to 375°F (190°C).

2. Cook quinoa according to package instructions.

3. In a large bowl, combine cooked quinoa, broccoli florets, shredded chicken, Greek yogurt, milk, shredded cheddar cheese, Dijon mustard, salt, and pepper.

4. Transfer the mixture to a greased baking dish.

5. If desired, sprinkle Panko breadcrumbs on top for added crunch.

6. Bake for 25-30 minutes until the casserole is bubbly and golden.

7. Allow it to cool slightly before serving.

13. Egg and Vegetable Breakfast Wrap

Ingredients:

- 2 large eggs, beaten

- 1 cup spinach leaves

- 1/2 cup cherry tomatoes, diced

- 1/4 cup feta cheese, crumbled

- 1 whole-grain or gluten-free wrap

- 1 teaspoon olive oil

- Salt and pepper to taste

- Avocado slices for topping

Instructions:

1. In a skillet, Increase the olive oil temperature over medium heat.

2. Add beaten eggs, spinach, cherry tomatoes, and feta cheese to the skillet.

3. Scramble the mixture until the eggs are cooked through.

4. Season with salt and pepper to make it sweet.

5. Spoon the egg and vegetable mixture onto the wrap.

6. Top with avocado slices before wrapping and serving.

14. Lentil and Vegetable Curry

Ingredients:

- 1 cup dried green or brown lentils, rinsed

- 1 onion, finely chopped

- 2 carrots, peeled and diced

- 1 bell pepper, diced

- 1 zucchini, sliced

- 1 can (14 oz) coconut milk

- 2 tablespoons curry powder

- 1 teaspoon turmeric

- 1 teaspoon cumin

- Salt and pepper to taste

- Fresh cilantro for garnish

- Cooked brown rice for serving

Instructions:

1. In a pot, combine lentils, chopped onion, diced carrots, bell pepper, sliced zucchini, coconut milk, curry powder, turmeric, cumin, salt, and pepper.

2. Bring the mixture to a boil, then reduce heat and simmer for 25-30 minutes until lentils are tender.

3. Adjust seasoning to taste.

4. Serve the lentil and vegetable curry over cooked brown rice.

5. Garnish with fresh cilantro before serving.

15. Greek Chicken Salad with Quinoa

Ingredients:

- 1 pound of grilled and sliced boneless, skinless chicken breasts

- 1 cup quinoa, cooked

- 1 cucumber, diced

- 1 cup cherry tomatoes, halved

- 1/2 red onion, thinly sliced

- 1/2 cup Kalamata olives, pitted and sliced

- 1/2 cup crumbled feta cheese

- 2 tablespoons olive oil

- Juice of 1 lemon

- 1 teaspoon dried oregano

- Salt and pepper to taste

Instructions:

1. In a large bowl, combine grilled and sliced chicken, cooked quinoa, diced cucumber, cherry tomatoes, sliced red onion, Kalamata olives, and crumbled feta cheese.

2. In a small bowl, whisk together olive oil, lemon juice, dried oregano, salt, and pepper to make the dressing.

3. Drizzle the dressing over the salad and toss to combine.

4. Serve the Greek chicken salad with quinoa as a refreshing and protein-packed meal.

16. Salmon and Asparagus Foil Packets

Ingredients:

- 4 salmon fillets

- 1 bunch asparagus, trimmed

- 2 tablespoons olive oil

- 2 cloves garlic, minced

- 1 lemon, sliced

- Fresh dill for garnish

- Salt and pepper to taste

Instructions:

1. Preheat the oven to 375°F (190°C).

2. Place each salmon fillet on a piece of foil.

3. Arrange asparagus around the salmon.

4. Drizzle olive oil over salmon and asparagus. Sprinkle minced garlic, salt, and pepper.

5. Place lemon slices on top of the salmon.

6. Seal the foil packets and bake in the oven for 15-20 minutes.

7. Garnish with fresh dill before serving.

17. Quinoa and Black Bean Salad with Avocado-Lime Dressing

Ingredients:

- 1 cup quinoa, cooked

- 1 can (15 oz) of drained and rinsed black beans,

- 1 cup of fresh or frozen corn kernels

- 1 red bell pepper, diced

- 1/4 cup red onion, finely chopped

- 1 avocado, diced

- Juice of 2 limes

- 2 tablespoons olive oil

- 1 teaspoon cumin

- Salt and pepper to taste

- Fresh cilantro for garnish

Instructions:

1. In a large bowl, combine cooked quinoa, black beans, corn, diced bell pepper, red onion, and diced avocado.

2. In a small bowl, whisk together lime juice, olive oil, cumin, salt, and pepper to make the dressing.

3. Drizzle the dressing over the salad and toss to combine.

4. Garnish with fresh cilantro before serving.

18. Turkey and Vegetable Skillet with Cauliflower Rice

Ingredients:

- 1 pound ground turkey

- 1 tablespoon olive oil

- 1 onion, diced

- 2 bell peppers, diced

- 1 zucchini, diced

- 2 cloves garlic, minced

- 1 can (14 oz) diced tomatoes

- 1 teaspoon Italian seasoning

- Salt and pepper to taste

- 4 cups cauliflower rice, cooked

- Fresh parsley for garnish

Instructions:

1. In a skillet, brown ground turkey over medium heat. Set aside.

2. In the same skillet, heat olive oil and sauté diced onion, bell peppers, zucchini, and minced garlic until softened.

3. Add browned turkey back to the skillet and stir in diced tomatoes, Italian seasoning, salt, and pepper.

4. Simmer for 10-15 minutes until flavors meld.

5. Serve the turkey and vegetable skillet over cooked cauliflower rice.

6. Garnish with fresh parsley before serving.

19. Veggie-Packed Quinoa Bowl with Lemon-Tahini Dressing

Ingredients:

- 1 cup quinoa, cooked

- 1 cup broccoli florets, steamed

- 1/2 cup cherry tomatoes, halved

- 1/2 cup cucumber, diced

- 1/4 cup red bell pepper, diced

- 1/4 cup shredded carrots

- 2 tablespoons pumpkin seeds

- 2 tablespoons tahini

- Juice of 1 lemon

- 1 tablespoon olive oil

- 1 teaspoon honey (optional)

- Salt and pepper to taste

Instructions:

1. In a bowl, combine cooked quinoa, steamed broccoli, cherry tomatoes, cucumber, red bell pepper, shredded carrots, and pumpkin seeds.

2. In a small bowl, whisk together tahini, lemon juice, olive oil, honey (if using), salt, and pepper to make the dressing.

3. Drizzle the dressing over the quinoa bowl and toss to combine.

4. Serve the veggie-packed quinoa bowl as a nutrient-rich and flavorful meal.

20. Chicken and Vegetable Kabobs with Herb Marinade

Ingredients:

- 1 pound boneless, skinless chicken breasts, cut into cubes

- 1 zucchini, sliced

- 1 red onion, cut into wedges

- 1 bell pepper, diced

- 1/4 cup olive oil

- 2 tablespoons fresh herbs (rosemary, thyme, or oregano), chopped

- 2 cloves garlic, minced

- Juice of 1 lemon

- Salt and pepper to taste

- Wooden or metal skewers

Instructions:

1. In a bowl, combine cubed chicken, sliced zucchini, onion wedges, and diced bell pepper.

2. In a separate bowl, mix olive oil, fresh herbs, minced garlic, lemon juice, salt, and pepper to make the marinade.

3. Pour the marinade over the chicken and vegetables, ensuring they are well-coated. Let it soak for minimum of 30 minutes.

4. Thread chicken and vegetables onto skewers.

5. Grill the skewers on medium-high heat for 10-15 minutes or until chicken is cooked through and vegetables are tender.

6. Serve the chicken and vegetable kabobs as a delicious and protein-packed meal.

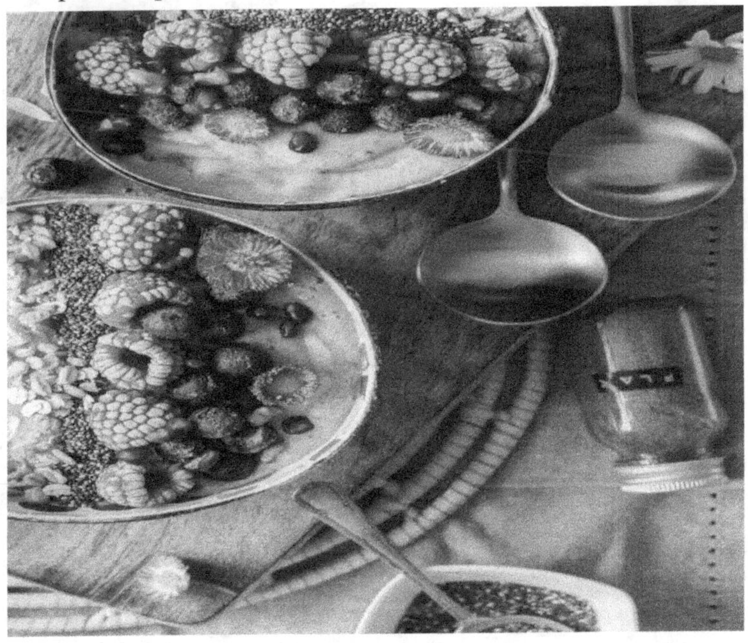

CONCLUSION

In concluding the Thyroid Cancer Diet Cookbook for Beginners, I invite readers to embark on a transformative journey towards better health.

Nourishing both the body and soul, this cookbook provides a rich tapestry of flavorful recipes meticulously crafted to support thyroid health.

From nutrient-packed salads to delectable mains, each dish is a testament to the synergy between taste and wellness. As we close the culinary chapters, remember that this cookbook is not just a collection of recipes but a guide to a vibrant and wholesome lifestyle.

May these nourishing creations empower you to savor not only the exquisite flavors but also the vitality that comes with embracing a thyroid-friendly diet.

Here's to your health, happiness, and a future filled with culinary delights that contribute to your overall well-being.

As you reach the final page of the Thyroid Cancer Diet Cookbook for Beginners, my heartfelt gratitude flows to everyone.

Thank you for embarking on this culinary journey towards thyroid health and overall well-being. May these recipes bring joy to your tables and vitality to your lives.

Your commitment to nourishing your body is a powerful step toward a healthier and happier you. Remember, the kitchen is not just a place for meals; it's a haven for self-care. Wishing you continual success on your path to good health.

With gratitude,

Patricia Camire

HAPPY COOKING!!!

www.ingramcontent.com/pod-product-compliance
Lightning Source LLC
Chambersburg PA
CBHW070744260726
48660CB00007B/2977